Ultimate Get In Shape Guide!

Weight Loss

Metabolism Secrets, Diet Tricks, And HIIT High Intensity Interval Training For Fast Fat Loss And To Build Muscle Fast!

I0428327

Sarah Brooks

STOP!!! Before you read any further....Would you like to know the Secrets of Body Transformation?

If your answer is yes, then you are not alone. Thousands of people are looking for the secret to rapidly burn body fat, keep the weight off, become healthier, and truly transform their body and life for good.

If you have been searching for these answers without much luck, you are in the right place!

Not only will you gain incredible insight in this book, but because I want to make sure to give you as much value as possible, right now for a limited time you can get full **100% FREE access to a VIP bonus EBook** entitled **THE 7 KEYS TO BODY TRANSFORMATION!**

Just Go Here For Free Instant Access:

www.liveFitVIP.com

Legal Notice

Disclaimer Notice

Table Of Contents

Introduction

I want to thank you and congratulate you for purchasing the book, *"Weight Loss!"*

This book contains proven steps and strategies on how to get in shape with HIIT and dieting.

Getting in shape is the combination of having the right knowledge, setting realistic goals and having the motivation to do it.

One aspect of a healthy lifestyle is committing to a healthy diet. Different types of diet can work for different people and the main key is to find one that fits your lifestyle. You also have to remember to get enough nutrients to make sure that you are performing at your maximum capacity.

You cannot get in shape without exercising. Humans are genetically designed to be active. HIIT exercise is an efficient and quick workout which you can do almost anywhere. You can also add other physical activities that you like.

This book also contains many tips on how you can stay motivated to reach your goal. Everyone gets discouraged at times but those who succeed always find a way to conquer challenges and achieve better results.

Thanks again for purchasing this book, I hope you enjoy it!

Chapter 1: The Main Reason Most People Never Get In Shape

Committing to a healthy lifestyle can be difficult most especially for people who have never considered it before. It is easy to find a reason to skip workouts and keep on eating junk food all the time.

Here are the top reasons why most people never get in shape:

Busy schedule

People who have a rigid work schedule may reason that they cannot find enough time to exercise. However, unless you work for 16 hours a day seven days in a week, most people can squeeze in 30 minutes of exercise a day. You can even take few minutes break from work every few hours to walk or stretch in place.

If you do not have enough time, you can break up your workout routine into shorter sessions. Remember that having a little bit of workout is better than none at all. Also, people who are really committed to healthy lifestyle find time to work out no matter their work schedule.

Low energy

After a day's work, some prefer to relax at home and watch TV instead of working out. Exercise actually gives people more energy and increases their stamina. Working out triggers the production of endorphin which can make you feel good and also improves better blood circulation.

You can also exercise first thing in the morning before you find excuse to skip it later. Again, you don't have to do a vigorous workout. You can simply jog for half an hour whenever you feel best.

Family responsibilities

Taking care of your children can take a toll on your schedule but it is not an excuse to stop working out. Taking your children in the park can be both fun and functional. You can spend time playing with them and exercise at the same time. There are a lot of activities you can enjoy with your kids like running or riding a bike around the neighborhood. Also, you will be setting a good example for your children if they see their parents living a healthy and active lifestyle.

Boring exercise

The best way to combat boredom is to find an activity that you enjoy. There are a lot of exercises that can fit any preference and personality. You should also switch up your routine every few months to avoid losing motivation. You can also enlist some friends or join a group to have more motivation.

Unhealthy diet

A person can commit to an exercise routine but they won't be able to get in shape if they do not change their unhealthy diet. Although not all diets can suit everybody, there is always a diet principle that can fit your lifestyle. All you have to do is to research and find it. Eating a balanced diet from carbohydrates, protein and fat is a good start. Remember that a healthy lifestyle is composed of healthy eating and enough exercise.

Tried before

Most people have tried to get in shape once or twice in their life. Some people succeed in their fitness goal while others fail. Those who fail might lose their motivation and decide not to try again. Set smaller and realistic goals next time. This way when you succeed in your goal, you are more motivated to accomplish another one.

Chapter 2: Flexible Dieting, Low Carb, Intermittent Fasting - How To Know What Works, And More Importantly, What Will Work For You!

It does not matter how scientifically sound a diet is or how many people have succeeded in it. What is important is that the diet works for you and that you can maintain it for a lifetime.

Tips in finding the right diet for you

- The diet plan should fit your lifestyle. Look for the diet that encourages you to eat the way you prefer to eat.
- Find a diet that can match your exercise level. Some diet plans encourage you to get moderate exercise while others propose rigorous exercise. If you are not very active, a plan that requires several hours at the gym everyday may not be suitable for you. Choose a program that can include exercise which you can do on a regular basis.
- You can stick with the diet forever. You should choose a diet that you can follow for the rest of your life. If your goal is only to lose the weight and then stop once you achieved your goal, you will most likely gain the weight back.
- Consider your time and budget. Some plans may include meal replacements which can work for busy people while others may prefer to cook their own food. You should also choose food that can fit your budget.
- Consider how quickly you can lose the weight. Seeing fast results can be a great motivator but make sure that you do not gain the weight back by sticking to the diet.
- The best weight loss plan is the one that corrects your unhealthy habits and does not make you feel like you're on a rigid 'diet' phase. Going on a diet can trigger cravings and frustration if you do not get your goal. Look for a plan that can help you tailor a healthy lifestyle.
- Some plans contain a long list of foods to avoid. This can lead to cravings and binges but some people actually do better if they totally eliminate their trigger foods. If you cannot totally avoid certain foods then you have to find a plan that allows small portions of these foods. Studies also

show that most people succeed by allowing room for indulges.

Flexible dieting

Flexible dieting does not follow a set of rigid and unsustainable rules. Here are the basic elements in flexible dieting.

Modification

People are given the liberty to eat the food that they enjoy. Foods are not labeled as bad or good. The diet encourages a well rounded diet where you can enjoy the food you like in moderation to accomplish your fitness goal.

If you have a medical condition that can be aggravated by eating particular food, then you should definitely avoid them. It should also be noted that the restrictions that you place on your eating habit should enable you to reach your goal.

Modify your diet based in your preferences then take into account what your medical restrictions are.

No guilty feeling

According to the flexible diet, people should be able to enjoy food without feeling guilty about it. There is also no reason to keep on eating the same food every day.

Most people who try to restrict too much components on their diet end up unhappy and can binge on it later. In most cases, your fat loss diet is the same as your regular diet.

Stick to the diet

Everyone experienced overeating at some point in their lives. The only thing that separates those who succeed and those who fail is what they do afterwards. The most ideal thing to do is to return to your diet and stay calm as possible. Flexible dieters also place things into perspective. They know that one scoop of ice cream or three cookies cannot make them gain weight immediately. Flexible dieters also set reasonable expectations from the beginning and were able to expect that there are some days where they will overeat.

Focus on maintaining fat loss

People who stick with a rigid diet can only do it if they focus on the short term goal. While you might reach your goal, maintaining it can be very difficult. Remember that your habits while you are still losing the weight are what enable you to keep the weight off as well.

Intermittent fasting

Studies have found that people who have significantly reduced their calorie consumption lived longer and healthier lives. There are different ways to fast and one method can work better for one person.

Leangains

This fasting method encourages people to fast for 14 hours for women and 16 hours for men. During this time, people are only allowed to consume black coffee with calorie free sweeteners. The next few hours are their feeding time. What people eat depends on whether they will be working out. People who exercise should consume more carbohydrates while fat intake should be higher during rest days. Protein consumption should be high every day.

Eat stop eat

In this method, people are advised to fast for 24 hours in a week. During this time, you are not allowed to eat anything but can consume calories free beverages. You can go back to your normal diet after the 24 hours. The main idea for this is to reduce you overall calorie intake without limiting any type of food. Resistance training is also an important factor in this plan.

Warrior diet

People in this diet are expected to fast for 20 hours then eat one large meal at night. People are encouraged to eat only small meal portions during the 20 hours of fasting and consume few servings of fresh juice and fruits. During the four hours, you can eat vegetables, protein and fat in that specific order. You are only allowed to eat carbohydrates if you still feel hungry after eating dinner.

Fat loss forever

You get one cheat day per week which is followed by a 36 hour fasting. The rest of the week is split into different fasting schedules. The longest fasts are done during your busiest days which allow you to avoid hunger pains and focus on being productive instead.

UpDay DownDay

This diet encourages people to eat very little on one day and eat normal the next. On the fast day, people are encouraged to eat around 400-500 calories only. The founders of this diet recommend meal replacement shakes during your diet days to ensure that you are still getting the essential nutrients that your body needs. The next day, you can eat normally.

Low carb diets

Low carbohydrate diets are one of the oldest diets in the world. It is based in a principle that reduction in carbohydrate consumption can decrease the body's insulin production and result in fat loss. The main idea of low carbohydrate diet is to force the body to use fat as its main fuel.

People are attracted to low carbohydrates because it leads to rapid weight loss. Celebrities go on a low carbohydrate diet because they need to drop weight for a film and not as a way for permanent lifestyle.

Chapter 3: Superfoods That Boost Your Metabolism And Burn More Calories

A person's metabolism is one of the key factors in losing and maintaining weight. Here are some of the foods that can boost your metabolism naturally.

Egg whites

Egg whites contain balanced amino acids which can keep your metabolism working. Eggs also contain a lot of vitamins and protein which can fill you up during the day.

Lean meat

Lean meat is rich in iron and contains enough minerals that can combat slow metabolism. Try to eat three servings of iron rich food daily.

Chili peppers

Chili peppers contain capsaicin which can increase your metabolism right after eating it. You can include a teaspoon of chopped chili peppers into your meals every day. Chili pepper is also rich in Vitamin C.

Coffee

Studies show that people who drank coffee had 16 percent higher metabolism than those that do not drink coffee.

Citrus fruits

Citrus fruits are rich in vitamin C which can metabolize fat faster and help you lose weight. Increasing your daily intake of vitamin C can boost your fat burning potential by 39%.

Berries

Berries are high in fiber. The body cannot digest fiber but it can burn calories while trying to digest it. Berries are also relatively low in calories and high in vitamins. Fiber also bond with the fat in the intestine and eliminate them through the digestive tract.

Garlic

Garlic is a super food that can boost your immunity and prevent diseases. Adding garlic into your meals can increase the amount of calories burned during the day and help decrease fat production.

Green tea

While this is technically a drink and not a food, green tea can also increase your metabolism because it contains EGCG which promotes fat burn.

Chapter 4: 20 Diet Tricks For Faster Weight Loss

While the concept of weight loss can be easy to understand, not everyone is capable of losing as much weight as they want.

Here are some tips in losing weight fast:

- Food diary. Keeping a food diary can make you aware of the amount of food you consume. This can also make you more conscious about your food choices.
- Enlist a weight loss buddy. Having a support system can help you stick with your weight loss program. This can also make you more accountable for your actions.
- Make your own mantra. Repeating positive thoughts or mantra during the day can help reinforce positive outlook in your life.
- Watch what you drink. One way to cut 300 calories in your diet is swapping soda and other sweetened beverage with water instead. Also, these drinks do not give you any sense of fullness like food.
- Chew slowly. Chewing slowly enables you to enjoy your food better. It also gives your stomach enough time to gauge your hunger level. If you eat slowly, you might discover that you don't need that much food to satisfy your hunger.
- Drink water when you feel like eating. Thirst can be mistaken for hunger so try to drink water and decide whether you are truly hungry or just thirsty.
- Sniff banana, apple or peppermint. Studies show that sniffing your food tricks the brain that you are actually eating it.
- Eat in front of mirrors. Studies show that people who ate in front of mirrors reduced their calories by one third. Looking at yourself while eating can remind you of your goals.
- Eat whole foods. Eat whole fruits and vegetables. They do not contain any artificial ingredient and have vitamins and minerals.
- Walk before dinner. Walking for few minutes before dinner can help you burn calories and reduce your appetite in the process.

- Put less food on your plate. The more food you place on your plate, the more likely you are to overeat. Cut down your servings by one third and only go for seconds if you are still hungry.
- Eat 90% of your meals at home. You are more likely to control your portions when you are home. Restaurants also have relatively large servings.
- Order the small portion. Ordering the smallest take out can limit the total amount of calories that you consume. This is also a good principle to apply on your cheat day.
- Eat water rich food. Foods that have high water content can fill your stomach up without too much calories. Foods that have high water content are zucchini, cucumbers and tomatoes.
- Bulk up your meals with vegetables. Adding vegetables to any of your meals instantly bulks it up without adding too much calories. It also adds more flavor and variety.
- Try to avoid white foods. White foods like white bread, potatoes and rice contain simple carbohydrates that can cause blood sugar spikes. Replace it with the whole wheat variety instead.
- Switch to regular coffee. Fancy coffee bought at coffee shops are loaded with added sugar and other ingredients that increases its calories. Invest in good coffee beans since it tastes just as great.
- Eat cereals for breakfast five days in a week. Studies show that people who consume cereal for breakfast are less likely to be obese since it contains fiber and calcium.
- Try hot sauce and Cajun seasonings. These seasonings pack a lot of flavor with just few calories. They can also improve your digestion and increase your metabolism temporarily.
- Eat most of your meals before noon. Studies show that the more you eat during the first half of the day, the less likely you are to eat in the evening.

Chapter 5: An Introduction To HIIT High Intensity Interval Training

HIIT or High Intensity Interval Training has been dubbed as the best way to burn fat and increase cardiovascular fitness in a short amount of time. The main idea is to exercise at you maximum capacity for a minute followed by an active rest for 30 seconds. This keeps your body moving and your heart rate up. Most experts recommend HIIT workouts two to three times in a week.

Benefits of HIIT

Efficient

HIIT is very efficient that it is mostly recommended for people with busy schedule. Researches show that 2 weeks of HIIT can improve your aerobic fitness as much as 6-week endurance training.

Burns more fat

Because of the energy required to perform HIIT exercises, you can burn a lot of calories in a short amount of time. You also burn more fat 24 hours after your work out compared to a regular workout.

Healthier heart

HIIT enables people to strengthen their heart. People who incorporated HIIT into their lifestyle were able to perform more activities at a longer time compared to when they first started.

No equipment necessary

Any plyometric exercise can be part of HIIT workout. This enables you to exercise anywhere and anytime.

Loss fat and not muscle

People who have tried to lose weight know that it is difficult to lose fat without muscle as well. HIIT allows you to preserve your muscles while losing fat.

Increase metabolism

HIIT stimulates human growth hormone which can increase your metabolism and even slow your ageing process.

Up for the challenge

HIIT is not a workout that you can do half-heartedly. Since it is so short, you will be required to work hard the whole time. This is ideal for people who do not like boring workouts.

Chapter 6: The Science Behind HIIT Training And Why It Burns Fat Faster In Less Time

Compelling research and studies show that short burs of intensive workout is the ideal form of exercise. Not only is it a more effective cardio exercise but it also provides other benefits like a boost in human growth hormone that you cannot get on a regular exercise.

HIIT vs. endurance training

Endurance training like a marathon event requires you to perform low intensity activities to last for a longer period of time. This requires aerobic energy that is sustained by oxygen. Oxygen breaks down the carbohydrates and fats. In high intensity exercise, you are using your anaerobic metabolism that does not involve oxygen. This burns more calories since your body struggles to keep up with the activity.

In HIIT, you are using two energy systems. You would spend short period of time doing a high intensity exercise followed by an active rest. The work is primarily done during the high intensity phase and muscles recover during the break.

Studies

One of the earliest studies for HIIT was conducted in Laval University in Canada. One group followed a 15 day program of HIIT while others performed steady cardio for 20 weeks. While those that followed traditional cardio burned 15,000 more calories than the HIIT group, people who followed the HIIT program lost more body fat.

Another study in East Tennessee State University also had the same results with the subjects loosing 2% of body fat in 8 weeks. The subjects that followed traditional cardio lost no body fat.

Scientist believes that the main reason that it can burn fat more effectively is because of its effect in the metabolism. A study in Baylor College of Medicine found out the people who performed HIIT burned more calories in the next 24 hours of their workout than endurance trainees. HIIT is difficult for the body so it requires more energy to keep up with the activity.

Research confirmation

Various researches also prove that HIIT can stop fat production. People who practiced HIIT have higher muscle fibers for fat oxidation. You can effectively increase your fat oxidation by 30% in just two weeks of HIIT workout. As an additional benefit, researches also conclude that short exercise sessions also allow you to retain your muscle mass.

Chapter 7: HIIT Workout Routines For Beginners

It is important to strategically increase your workout intensity as you start to incorporate HIIT workouts in your fitness routine. Do not attempt difficult exercises immediately most especially if you have not been physically active for the past months. Here are some workout routines for beginners which lasts for 10 minutes or even less. Since these workouts are relatively low impact, you can perform it every day. Aim to stay in the beginner phase for at least 2 weeks.

Treadmill HIIT

You can incorporate HIIT workout into your regular gym session. This workout changes both the incline and pace to keep your body challenged.

2 minutes of brisk walk on a 3.0 incline

2 minutes slow jogging on 1.5 incline

1 minute run on 1.5 incline

2 minutes walk on 3.5 inline

2 minutes slow jogging on 3.5 inline

1 minute sprint on 3.5 inline

Indoor HIIT

You can also workout at home. This routine does not require any equipment so feel free to do it anytime and anywhere. Remember to rest for 30 seconds between each exercise.

10 lunge jumps for 1 minute

20 pushups in 1.5 minutes

30 squats in 1.5 minutes

40 chair dips in 1.5 minute

50 mountain climbers in 2 minutes

Outdoor HIIT

Exercising outdoors can have psychological benefits. If the weather permits, take your workout outdoors and take advantage of the natural setting.

- Park bench

1 minute slow jogging

30 seconds sprint

20 leg step ups

20 triceps dips

20 squat jumps

2 minutes active rest

- Railing

1 min jogging

30 seconds sprint

10 incline lever pull-ups

30 pile squat jumps

Chapter 8: HIIT Workout Routines For Intermediates

After two weeks of performing easy 10 minute HIIT routines, you can begin lengthening your workouts and include more challenging exercises. It is recommended to use a timer for these exercises and try to do as many as you can within the given amount of time. Repeat the routine 3 times with 30 seconds of rest between exercise and 2 minutes of active rest between sets. You can perform this exercise 3-4 times in a week.

Warm up:

Jog for a minute

Jumping jacks for a minute

HIIT workout:

Speed skater for 45 seconds

Stand with your feet apart. Bend the right knee and extend the left leg into a lunge position. Lower your body to stretch the left leg then shift your weight to the right leg and lunge.

Jump free burpees for 45 seconds

Stand with your hands over your head. Push hips back and place your palms flat on the floor in a plank position. Lower into a push up then push your body up into a squat. Stand up and return to the starting position.

Seated Tuck jumps for 45 seconds

Sit on a chair with your back leaning slightly. Engage your core and bend your knees at 90 degrees. Point the toes on the floor. Lift both your knees and sit upright as you pull your legs up.

Kicking plant for 45 seconds

Begin in a plank position. Jump into a squat position while kicking the left leg towards the right while your right hand reaches towards your left foot. Return to plank position and repeat on the other side.

Butterfly squats for 45 seconds

Start in a squat position with one of your hand on top of the other. Quickly stand up and reach your hands overhead while lifting your heels off the floor. Return to the squat position as fast as you can.

Rising lunge for 45 seconds

Lunge with your left leg bent and right leg in front. Hold your hands in a fist on your side. Stand up and extend your hands overhead. Keep your feet in position throughout the movement.

Chapter 9: HIIT Workout Routines For Experts

By this time, your body is already be used to HIIT workout. This routine is longer and much more difficult. It also targets most of your muscles which make it a good total body work out.

Round 1:

- Burpees

Bend your knees and place your hands on the floor. Jump back and place feet into a plank position. Push your body up and then stand.

- Mountain climbers

Start in a plank position. Lift your knees towards your stomach in a climbing motion. Repeat it with the other leg.

- Jumping jacks

Stand with your feet close together. Jump up and spread your legs and extend your arms overhead. Jump up and place feet together.

Complete three circuits: 10 repetitions for the first round, 15 for the second and 20 for the last round.

- Jump rope for 3 minutes
- Rest for 1 minute

Round 2:

- Walking lunges

Stand with your feet apart. Place hands on your hips. Step one leg forward while bending knees until it almost touches the ground. Extend both knees to push your body back up. Repeat the lunge on the opposite leg.

- Inchworms

Stand with your feet apart. Bend until your hands touch the floor. Your body should look like an inverted V. Keep your core tight and walk forward with your hands. Lift your hips and walk your legs in.

- Lunge jumps

Stand with your feet together and lunge forward with the right leg. Jump straight and push your hands in the air. Switch your legs mid air and land in a lunge position with the left leg.

Complete three circuits: 30 seconds per exercise with 10 second break in between.

- Jump rope for 3 minutes
- Rest for 1 minute

Round 3:

- Squats

Place feet on the ground with your toes pointing outwards. Push your buttocks out and lower your chest to your knees.

- Pull-ups

Grab the bar with both of your hands facing away from you. Let your body hang down. Pull yourself up until your chin is above the bar. Stay in the position for few seconds then lower your body.

- Box jumps

Stand with your feet apart in the box. Drop your body into a quarter-squat position and jump back down. Try to land as quietly as possible.

- Skier jumps

Stand with your feet together. In a fast motion step, wide step to your right while bending the upper body at the waist. Make sure to balance your right foot and keep your left foot behind you. Repeat the movements on the other side.

Complete three circuits: 40 seconds each with 15 seconds rest in between

- Jump rope for 3 minutes
- Rest for 1 minute

Chapter 10: 20 Tips To Keep Motivation Sky High And Reach Your Fitness Goals

Being consistent is the key in achieving a good body. Here are some tips in staying motivated to reach your goal.

- Do not forget to have fun. Exercise should be a fun activity. The right mindset can get you through your first marathon or a difficult obstacle race.
- One hour of exercise is just 4% of your day. There are a lot of ways to incorporate exercise into your routine and one hour of physical activity is really not that much.
- Just walk. Studies show that women who walked 500 more steps in a day lost quarter of inch from their waist in 3 months.
- Try something new. Doing the same routine over and over again can get boring. Do not be afraid to try new workouts and you might find something you like.
- Remember the main reason why you are trying to get fit. Sometimes the best motivation knows the reason why you want to be fit in the first place whether it is to improve your health or to boost your self confidence.
- You're doing your body a favor. Working out should never feel like you're punishing yourself. On the contrary, think as if you are giving your body what it needs.
- Think like a champion. Set yourself up for success. Entertaining negative thoughts can make you fail. Believe in yourself and what you're capable of.
- Part of your life. Schedule your workouts as a normal part of your daily activities and avoid making excuses.
- Write it down. Studies show that seeing your goals in paper can keep you motivated. It also serves as a reminder of the things that you should be doing.
- Make it social. Exercise is fun if you do it with your friends. Invite other people on a walk or attend a dance class and use it as an opportunity to socialize.
- Reward yourself. Fitness is the main reward of a healthy lifestyle but you can also motivate yourself by treating yourself with some small rewards like new clothes or shoes.

- Know when to rest. Be flexible in your workouts. You also need to rest to give your body enough time to recover.
- Strive for progress and not perfection. Even if you are only seeing slow results, remember that it is better than not improving at all. You can also look back to when you first started and how far you have come.
- Find motivation in others. You can find several inspiring fitness stories everywhere. Remember that if they can do it, so can you.
- Stress relief. One of the best benefits of working out is the reduction in stress immediately afterwards. Some people also swear that exercise can help them stay calm throughout the day.
- Look for challenges. Running your first half-marathon can both be challenging and exciting. Finishing the race can empower you and keep you motivated to continue on your fitness journey.
- Avoid regret. If you constantly make excuses, you will also feel the regret afterwards. The only bad workout is the one that you didn't do.
- Other look up to you. Whether you broadcast your fitness journey or silently work through it, people will notice the change in you. The change in your lifestyle can have a great effect on other people as well. You could be setting a good example for your family and friends.
- Good comments. You will feel good once you start to receive compliments from other people about your progress. Knowing that other people also appreciate your progress can be greatly motivating.
- Music. Good workout music can be all you need to stay motivated in your workout. Listening to your favorite tunes can also keep your energy high.

Conclusion

Thank you again for purchasing this book on weight loss!

I am extremely excited to pass this information along to you, and I am so happy that you now have read and can hopefully implement these strategies going forward.

I hope this book was able to help you understand different diets as well as the concept of HIIT and how to incorporate it in your daily routine.

The next step is to get started using this information and to hopefully live a healthy and productive life!

Please don't be someone who just reads this information and doesn't apply it, the strategies in this book will only benefit you if you use them!

If you know of anyone else that could benefit from the information presented here, please inform them of this book.

Finally, if you enjoyed this book and feel it has added value to your life in any way, please take the time to share your thoughts and post a review on Amazon. It'd be greatly appreciated!

Thank you and good luck!

Preview Of:

<u>Natural Remedies!</u>

Natural Herbal Remedies And Beyond For Your Health And Natural Beauty!

Introduction

I want to thank you and congratulate you for purchasing the book, *"Natural Remedies! - Natural Herbal Remedies And Beyond For Your Health And Natural Beauty!"*

This book contains insight to the amazing world of natural herbal remedies and how incredible they can be for your health!

This day and age many people automatically turn to the traditional medical field for all of their health and beauty problems looking for the answers. Unfortunately, many times these solutions can also come with their own problems. Now you have two problems to be treated! The first one you were looking to take care and a myriad of other side effects you must now also treat.

Over the years I have begun to realize that this is a very common and many people are looking for additional, more holistic ways of treating minor issues that won't have them second guessing later. This is my motivation for creating this book and hope you will find many solutions to everyday problems, and live a much healthier and happy life!

Thanks again for purchasing this book, I hope you enjoy it!

Chapter 1: Natural Herbal Remedies: An Introduction

I am so happy you have decided to go down this journey with me and I hope you find what you are looking for! I want to take a moment to explain why I have structured this book in the way it is. First this book is meant to provide you with as much information with as little clutter as possible, because at the end of the day what you want is solutions to your problems, not some fancy way of saying it! So please don't get hung up if you feel that sometimes the text is just giving you the facts and not a lot of fluff that is the way it is designed - so you can get the most out of it! Now let's get started!!!

What's so great about using natural remedies, you ask? There are many great things about it, often overlooked by people who are quite used to taking medication that's been prescribed to them or ones that they are most familiar with. There's nothing wrong with that, of course, but one needs to be mindful of the different side-effects that these chemicals may bring about. Many people turn to the use of these natural remedies (otherwise known as home remedies or folk medicine) for many of their ailments because of the fact that these are made out of natural ingredients. Herbs, vegetables and fruits are just a few of the most common ingredients used in these remedies. The best bit, however, is that many of these things can be easily found in an average kitchen.

But will it work? Well, if you consider the fact that throughout history people have used and relied upon these natural medicines, then the answer would be a solid yes. This was before modern medicine was invented and the use of synthetic drugs was propagated. It works but as to what extent, well, that varies from one individual to the next. For simple cures, however, even some doctors recommend their use instead of depending on over the counter medicine. Even in the food that we consume on a daily basis, there are healing properties that can help combat certain types of illnesses. It would be to our benefit if we harnessed it and used to as supplements to the medications that we're taking. In fact, if it happens to be potent enough, you can use it by itself. Research and studies do prove that many of these natural remedies possess properties that work in the same manner as synthetic medication.

How do you get started with it then? Well, first off, you would require a certain knowledge of which ingredients you need for a particular ailment. That's where this book is going to come in handy. We'll get more into the specifics later.

Spices, herbs and even fresh food can be used effectively when it comes to treating most ailments that can range from minor pains to even infections. These days, people would rely on antibiotics for these things. Those can be quite expensive, let's be honest, and in some cases, they can also cause adverse side effects if misused. There's also the fact that these antibiotics also end up killing the good or beneficial flora and fauna in our bodies, thus making recovery time lengthier than usual. In worst case scenarios, they can backfire and actually damage our immune system. With natural home remedies, however, you can avoid all of that. Besides treating the infection itself, it also helps in strengthening our immune system which makes it more capable of defending itself from other ailments. We also recover better with it as it readily promotes mending and healing of various aches and pains, as well as burns and wounds.

Besides medicine, you can also make use of home remedies to make your own mouthwash and if you're really good, toothpaste. Some people go to the extent of creating medicinal soaps that allow them to avoid mass marketed ones that might contain ingredients that they're allergic to, don't support or extremely harsh for the skin.

It takes a bit more work to achieve these, but if you're really keen, a few hours out of your day should be enough. So, if you have certain skin issues and want to give natural soap a try, look to the later chapters for instructions on how you can make some. Besides hygiene products, you might also want to try creating remedies for indigestion and constipation, both common problems for modern man considering the diet we all have. This would be good if you need to regularly take something in order to be able to move your bowel easily.

What else can these home remedies be used for? There's also some that you can make in order to help yourself or a loved one recover from the flu in a quicker fashion. You may also make teas that would help relieve a cough or a sore throat. A throat spray (typically used for asthma) can also be made through the use of natural ingredients that, when compared to a store-bought one, would be far cheaper.

We've already touched on it but these remedies aren't just meant for internal use only. Besides the soaps and the mouthwash, you can also create your own natural cleanser that would treat skin conditions such as acne. An antiseptic spray made from natural ingredients can also be concocted and this would be great for eliminating dermatitis, as well as killing bacteria from scratches or cuts. It can also effectively heal blisters.

Needless to say, there is a lot that one can do when it comes to home remedies. All you really need is a simple guide, as well as a few free hours for research. The more familiar you are with the benefits of a particular ingredient, the better you will be at making and mixing remedies.

Thanks for Previewing My Exciting Book Entitled:

"Natural Remedies: Natural Herbal Remedies And Beyond For Your Health And Natural Beauty!"

To purchase this book, simply go to the Amazon Kindle store and simply search:

"NATURAL REMEDIES"

Then just scroll down until you see my book. You will know it is mine because you will see my name "Sarah Brooks" underneath the title.

Alternatively, you can visit my author page on Amazon to see this book and other work I have done. Thanks so much, and please don't forget your free bonuses

DON'T LEAVE YET! - CHECK OUT YOUR FREE BONUSES BELOW!

Free Bonus Offer: Get Free Access To The www.LiveFitVIP.com VIP Newsletter!

Once you enter your email address you will immediately get free access to this awesome newsletter!

But wait, right now if you join now for free you will also get free access to the "The 7 Keys To Body Transformation" free EBook!

To claim both your FREE VIP NEWSLETTER MEMBERSHIP and your FREE BONUS eBook on THE 7 KEYS TO BODY TRANSFORMATION!

Just Go To:

www.liveFitVIP.com

www.ingramcontent.com/pod-product-compliance
Lightning Source LLC
Chambersburg PA
CBHW070938290526
45795CB00003B/1056